The Big Secret, Incontinence

The Big Secret, Incontinence

Sophia Kangarlu, M.D.
Anita Kangarlu

To my lovely daughter Chloe, who is an awesome writer
and is my inspiration.

To order additional copies of this book, contact:
Xlibris Corporation
1-888-795-4274
www.Xlibris.com
Orders@Xlibris.com
45551

Contents

Introduction

The Big Secret

Incontinence is one of the biggest secrets of our time. More than 25 million Americans suffer from some form of incontinence.

Incontinence affects all aspects of our life. It affects the location of the vacation, the job, the social gatherings, the finances, the color of our clothing, even our movements. It affects our food, our drink, sleep and rest, the time of laughter, and virtually all aspects of life. But still we do not hear anything about it in the media, not between people, not between doctors and patients, and not between husbands and wives.

Everybody is so embarrassed about incontinence that they do not want to talk about it and usually neglect it, and by negligence, most of the time, it becomes worse and decreases the quality of life significantly. It causes men and women to isolate themselves and do behaviors that surprise others, and often loved ones resent them without knowing the real cause. People even cancel important social events of close friends because of incontinence such as weddings, anniversaries, trips, and more.

Billions of dollars are spent; environment pollution is worsening, and the rate of depression and isolation increasing. People lose their independence and get transferred to nursing homes because of keeping this secret.

It is time the big secret comes out. We want to talk about it loud and clear. I plead to the media, to all women advocates, to all health advocates, to human rights advocates, to environmentalists, to all elderly advocates—let's break the silence many people suffered and are suffering still today. I plead to all women and men, at any age, to break the silence.

Do appropriate exercises at any age. These exercises are illustrated in this book. The accompanying DVD illustrates the exercises and can help you significantly reduce the incidence of incontinence.

I plead to all mothers and fathers to teach these exercises to your children. May the future generation be luckier and healthier than we are.

There is help out there. Just ask for it; do your part. Talk to your doctor.

One Woman's Story

Judy, a previously beautiful, energetic fifty-nine-year-old pharmaceutical rep, started noticing leakage when she was fifty-three, a few years after menopause. At first she started to avoid situations that caused leakage. Also, by using pads and frequent urinating, she was able to manage her job and the incontinence for up to two years. Then the amount of leakage got to be so much that hardly diapers could handle it. Preoccupied by the incontinence and mapping the bathrooms everywhere she went just added to the embarrassment, as well as the urine odor. She quit her job and tried to avoid many social events. She also tried to avoid physical activities causing urine loss and ended up in a very sedentary lifestyle and weight gain that worsened the condition altogether. She avoided intimacy with her husband as well, who was just confused by Judy's change of behavior.

Judy kept the big secret, and so nobody realized what was happening. Doctors suspected depression or early dementia as she never discussed the problem with any of her healthcare providers, and they simply never asked.

Incontinence changed Judy's life drastically. The quality of her life and others in her life was significantly reduced. Nobody knew the cause. She never told anyone—not her husband, her children, her friends, or her doctors. If only she knew there was help out there and she could benefit from it, maybe she and her husband and others in her life would have had a much better life.

Chapter One

When Incontinence Makes Life Miserable

1. Personal Problems

A. Social Isolation

Being embarrassed about accidents with incontinence is not something you should have to suffer. People with incontinence tend to isolate themselves from social events or public places in an attempt to hide their problem.

Incontinence makes traveling difficult because people fear having an accident and not being able to get to the restroom in time. Going to a party or social gathering becomes difficult for the same reasoning—fear of leakage. And if that isn't worry enough, a person with incontinence is constantly worried someone else will smell the odor of urine resulting from an accident.

When they do venture out to public places, most people with incontinence prefer seats or tables close to the restrooms in case there is an urgent need to rush to the toilet. This is embarrassing to discuss, even with their closest companions, children, or spouse. They are faced with constant worry of humiliation about their problem.

Most sufferers try to keep it a secret, but when they leak urine on furniture or their clothing, the secret is out. Then what? Will there be a place to change their clothes? Will they have to go home to clean up or cancel their plans? These are some of the problems incontinence brings out and can keep a person from attending weddings or having fun with friends at movies or gatherings. Since friends do not know about the real issue, they may be resentful of the mysterious behavior. Longtime relationships may break up. It all boils down to a very isolating lifestyle for the person with incontinence.

B. Sex

People with urinary incontinence usually have a more restricted sex life. One of the reasons is that most people usually don't communicate their problems and their fears. Some couples start sleeping separately because of the urine smell and fear of leakage. Leaking urine during sexual intercourse can be very stressful. Incontinence during orgasm, such as bed-wetting and loss of urine or fecal control, causes people to end most pleasurable sexual contact.

C. Travel

Toilet mapping becomes a habit of people with incontinence. In fact, people who once were very active traveling now look at each route as a milestone to get to the next bathroom. Some people with incontinence will avoid travel altogether. If they do go traveling, they must spend the time to find accommodations that have appropriate toilet access.

While traveling, men are more concerned about urinary accidents on the journey or in bed, while women are most concerned about the availability of bathrooms. Because of fear of a leakage accident, some people do not drink enough water while traveling and become dehydrated. Irritation of concentrated urine causes more leakage and incidents.

D. Effects on the Family

Most families have at least one member that is somehow affected by incontinence. The loss of dignity associated with incontinence makes personality changes in an individual that is usually bothersome to other family members.

The percentage of depression in incontinent adults is significantly higher as well. Incontinent adults develop psychological and physical problems that handling these issues is very difficult for other members of the family.

Economic issues associated with incontinence can have a significant burden on other family members. Incontinence is number 1 reason for nursing home placement. Many elderly people try to hide it to avoid placement by family members.

Chapter Two

What is Urinary Incontinence?

Urinary incontinence is the inability to hold urine and an uncontrollable loss of urine. It ranges between occasional leakages to frequent self-wetting. If urinary loss is causing negative effects on quality of life, usually diagnosis of urinary incontinence applies. In other words, urinary incontinence is involuntary loss of urine, which causes hygienic, personal, and social problems.

If you have the following symptoms, then you have urinary incontinence:

1. Involuntary urine loss.
2. Urine loss makes negative effect on quality of your life.
3. The leakage is objectively demonstrable.

It is very important to note that urinary incontinence is a medical condition and is not a part of aging or childbirth. Urinary incontinence can be treated and controlled like many other diseases and medical conditions.

You may have symptoms of urinary incontinence such as:

- Involuntary loss of urine during physical activity, laughing, coughing, etc., as seen in stress incontinence
- Involuntary loss of urine associated with strong desire to void, as seen in urge incontinence
- Urinary leakage in absence of urgency and without consciously knowing the urine loss, as in unconscious incontinence
- Involuntary loss of urine during sleep, as seen in nocturnal enuresis
- ontinuous incontinence

Types of Urinary Incontinence

1. Stress Incontinence

Involuntary loss of urine associated with coughing, sneezing, or even minimal activity, such as walking. Usually happens in multiparous women and worsened by lifting, straining, aerobic exercises, and constipation. Stress incontinence accounts for about 50% of cases.

How many times have you coughed or sneezed and wet your pants?

You could leak urine while you are walking on a treadmill at the gym even. Sometimes it's as simple as a walk around the block, or planting flowers in the yard even can induce incontinence.

Any rise in abdominal pressure can cause more pressure on the neck of your bladder. This is very common among young and middle-aged women. It is also very common for this age group to experience weakness of the urinary sphincter and pelvic muscles caused by childbirth, pelvic surgery, or abnormal position of urethra or uterus.

The name *stress incontinence* implies that the pressure of the laugh or sneeze increase the pressure in the abdomen that pushes on the bladder and urethra and consequently the urethra opens and urine leaks even if you may not have the urge to urinate.

Causes of Stress Urinary Incontinence

- Childbirth and pregnancy that causes weakening of the pelvic muscles and possibly damaging some nerves
- Smoking and chronic cough
  It causes continuous stress over abdomen, bladder, and urinary sphincter, and in time, leakage happens with minimal activity.
- In men, it is usually because of prostate surgery or hip fracture that causes damage to urethral sphincter.
- Obesity
  Extra weight causes stress and pressure over abdominal organs, bladder, and urethra and causes stress incontinence.

- Genetics and family history
  If you have a family history of stress urinary incontinence, it usually means weaker supporting tissue and weaker collagen, ligaments, and pelvic musculature. You may inherit that. You may need to start strengthening your muscles earlier.
- Menopause and hormonal changes
  In postmenopausal women, hormonal changes can reduce the urethra's resistance to urine flow. In addition, it causes decreased blood flow and thinning of tissue.

Most patients that suffer from stress incontinence find that getting out of bed in the morning can lead to an accident. In the morning, abdominal muscles push down on the bladder and cause pressure that can result in loss of urine. Usually, it is only a small amount, but bothersome all the same. Most people will live with this problem because it is a slight amount, but it leads to other loss of activity and a decrease in quality of life.

Patients may find that any increase in abdominal pressure starts an episode; they would discontinue that activity that causes a problem. So instead of getting up and exercising, they may become more sedentary. As this happens, their incontinence episodes increase.

In stress incontinence, you notice a range of severity. Minimal leakage is urine loss when you are laughing, coughing, or sneezing. Moderate leakage is when you lose urine when you do activities like standing, walking, or exercising. Sever incontinence is when you have urine loss just turning over in bed or switching sitting positions.

We will discuss the ways to prevent, delay, and treat stress incontinence in chapter XX in this book.

2. Urge Incontinence

If you have ever had a problem getting to the bathroom before having an accident, chances are you have urge incontinence. Incontinence because of overactive bladder is called urge incontinence.

Normally your bladder can hold about 6-12 ounces of urine, and you may urinate 6 or 7 times a day. But in urge incontinence, the sensation to urinate is so strong that you cannot reach the toilet in time.

Some people even leak urine upon washing their hands or washing dishes under running water or even hearing running water. An abrupt or intense urge to urinate cannot be suppressed before an accident happens.

One of the major problems patients with urge incontinence suffer is the inability to move quickly. If your mobility is challenged, getting to the bathroom can be a terrible hindrance. Urge incontinence is most commonly found in older patients with restricted movements that impede their way. It can present with no clear cause. It is most commonly found among residents who reside in nursing facilities.

Research indicates that a combination of overactivity of the muscles in the bladder (detrusor hyperactivity) with the inability to squeeze these muscles appropriately attribute to this condition. The inability to control these muscles may associate with brain disorders (especially stroke and dementia), which inhibit the nervous system's ability to control the bladder. The chronic overactivity of the bladder causes an intense urge to urinate regardless of whether it is day or night.

Some typical symptoms of overactive bladder include the following:

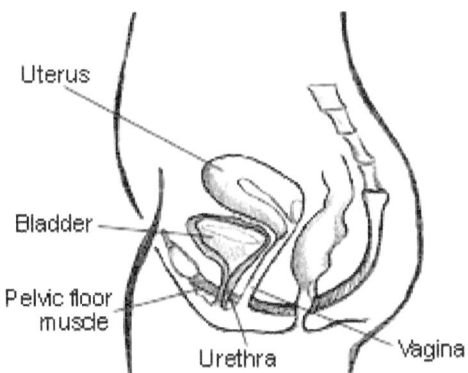

Female pelvic floor muscles

- Urinating more than eight times a day
- Strong and sudden desires to urinate
- Urinating more than three or four times during the night

With an overactive bladder, you may have a trigger event. One of the most common is referred to as key in the lock or garage door syndrome. These triggers occur when the patient tries to open a door. People who suffer from this condition usually have to urinate frequently and just cannot make it to the toilet on time. The patient reports urine just gushes out even though they may be losing only a small amount. The amount of urine can vary from minimal to severe.

Sleeping can be a problem for people with overactive bladder because either they need to get up to urinate or they will have accidents that awaken them. All aspects of life can begin to revolve around the bathroom.

Many patients develop behaviors to protect them from having accidents. One such behavior is to map out all the toilets in the places they will be going. This is called toilet mapping and is very common for someone with an overactive bladder.

Other behaviors are as follows:

- Repeatedly leaving important meetings because of frequent trips to bathroom
- Disturbed sleep and daytime irritability.
- Only sitting in the aisle seat of a plane or movies
- Wearing baggy or black clothing
- Withdrawal from sex to avoid embarrassment of urine leakage during sex
- Avoid some movements and some exercises not to be far from bathroom

3. Mixed Incontinence (having more than one type of incontinence)

Usually if you have more than one type of incontinence, you have mixed incontinence—usually a stress incontinence and urge incontinence combination. You would have signs and problems of both types, but one type is more bothersome.

For example, if you leak urine when you laugh or cough and also have a strong urge to urinate and leak urine before reaching the bathroom, you have mixed incontinence.

Most women with incontinence have mixed incontinence. Men after prostate surgery or prostate enlargement may develop mixed incontinence as well.

4. Overflow Incontinence

Dribbling most of the time without urge best describes how overflow incontinence affects a patient. You may feel like you cannot completely empty your bladder. Difficulty in starting to urinate is a significant problem. The problem lies in bladder emptying. The bladder cannot empty completely, so urine accumulates until it exceeds bladder capacity, forcing the urethral sphincter to open and urine to leak out.

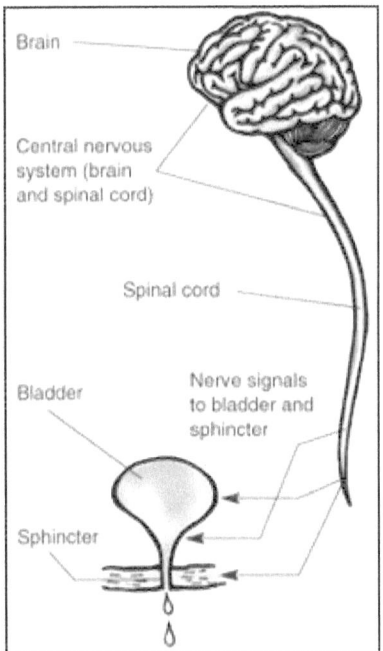

Nerves carry signals from the brain to the bladder and sphincter. Any disease, condition, or injury that damages nerves can lead to urination problems

Overflow incontinence has different causes. One of the most common causes is urethral blockage seen in prostate enlargement in men. The second important cause is weak bladder muscles to contract seen in neurological diseases or nerve damages. Nerve damage from diabetes mellitus, multiple sclerosis, herpes infection, injury of nerves during childbirth or postpartum vaginal tears can prevent bladder muscles from contracting effectively. Some medications that relax bladder muscles or make you unaware of the urge to urinate can cause overflow incontinence. Pelvic masses such as ovarian cysts or even a pregnant uterus can cause overflow incontinence. Abdominal and pelvic surgeries are among other causes.

Overflow incontinence can be a significant health problem. If bladder emptying is not treated, urine can go back to the kidneys and cause hydronephrosis and damage the kidney function. Men usually experience overflow incontinence because of prostate hypertrophy or a urethral stricture. If the prostate blocks the urethra, then the bladder does not empty completely during urination. Over-the-counter drugs like cold remedies can cause the urethral sphincter to close. Men who have some sort of obstruction will find they have a weak or poor stream of urine or that they have hesitancy in starting it. They may also have some post dribble all day long from the inability to empty their entire bladder. Some men report they have to strain just to urinate. Nerves carry signals from the brain to the bladder and sphincter. Any disease, condition, or injury that damages nerves can lead to urination problems.

In women, overflow incontinence usually happens when there is advanced pelvic prolapse, which can cause obstruction or kinking the bladder neck. Women feel as if their bladder is never empty, and they can dribble urine all day.

Constipation can be a major cause of overflow incontinence. Stool in the rectum can fill to the point of causing a large amount of pressure on the urethra and bladder neck.
If overflow incontinence is bothering you, please consult your physician. In some cases, urine can back up in the kidneys, which can lead to kidney damage. In addition, bladder infections can cause infections that are more serious.

5. Functional Incontinence

Functional incontinence is when you cannot reach a bathroom in time because of physical disability, obstacles, and problems in thinking or communicating that prevent a person from reaching a toilet. For example, a person with Alzheimer's disease may not think well enough to plan a trip to the bathroom in time or a person in a wheelchair may be blocked from getting to a toilet.

Most patients who have this type of incontinence demonstrate poor toileting habits, usually from a physical or mental inability to get to a toilet. Functional urinary incontinence is frequently misdiagnosed because the majority of patients have a normally functioning urinary tract. However, their mental or physical ability can affect when they go to the toilet on time.

Conditions that can affect those with functional incontinence include dementia, Parkinson's disease, Alzheimer's disease, spinal cord injuries, arthritis, and so many more. While some people might have problems with arthritis affecting their ability to undress and urinate, others with dementia are mentally incapable of making the decision to go to bathroom or even finding the bathroom.

Availability or closeness of restroom facilities can play an important part in functional incontinence. If the bathroom is too far away or is not equipped for the physically challenged, then the patient can be hindered from getting to the toilet on time.
Medications can also contribute to factors involving functional incontinence. Any medication that is a diuretic can cause frequent urinations in individuals who already have a problem getting to toilet facilities on time. Drugs that affect alertness, orientation, mobility, or dexterity can contribute to functional incontinence. In addition, these drugs can cause difficulty in communication with a caregiver to get the patient to the bathroom on time.

6. Reflex Incontinence

This type of incontinence is when there is no sensation and feeling to urinate. It is associated with patients who have birth defects or spinal cord injury and the nerve pathway between bladder and brain is damaged. Patients usually have advanced neurological impairment. Their bladder contracts without the urge or the sensation to void. This means they will urinate several times without sensation, therefore making it highly unpredictable when they need to get to a toilet.

Chapter Three

How the Urinary System Works

Micturition Cycle

During the storage phase, pressure remains low during filling, and eventually, there is a sense of imminent voiding. However, it is not an urgent sense. It is just a normal, natural sense that the bladder is getting full. There is no change in bladder pressure with that sensation. If it were a change in pressure and a sudden increase, it is an uninhibited bladder contraction or detrusor instability.

Normally, sensation occurs at low pressure without any change in pressure curve. Then you receive a normal desire to void and a sustained bladder contraction occurs with an increase in bladder pressure during the emptying phase with good relaxation of the urethra and complete emptying without residual urine volume. Then the bladder cycle fills again.

Innervations of the Lower Urinary Tract

Pudental nerve: Innervates pelvic floor and the voluntary sphincter of the urethra

Parasympathetic nervous system: The inputs coming from sacral area and pelvic nerves and provide parasympathetic input

Sympathetic nervous system: Important role in filling part and tighten the urethra with agonist action on urethral smooth muscles

Kidneys

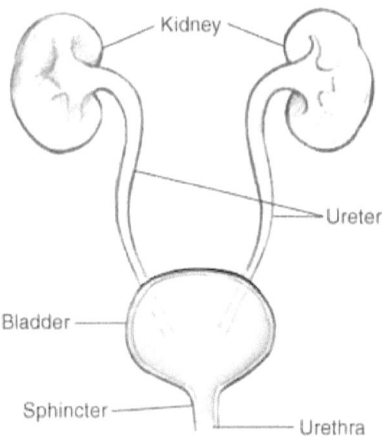

Kidneys are two beanlike organs that are located in the back on the sides of the spinal cord and in front of the lower rib cage. The kidney's function is to eliminate waste from the blood in the form of urine. Urine is constituted of 95% water and 5% waste materials. Urine travels from the kidneys through the ureters, which are approximately 9 inches long and collect into the urinary bladder.

Ureters are thin muscular tubes that connect kidney to bladder. Ureters pierce the bladder wall at an oblique angle and continue in the bladder wall for about 1 inch then they form the ureteral orifice. It is very important that during bladder contraction ureteral orifices pull down and in so ureters narrow down and urine does not go back to kidneys. If urine goes back to kidneys (vesicoureteral reflux) serious kidney damage can occur.

How the Bladder Works

The bladder is a hollow muscular sac behind pelvic bones. The bladder has an inner lining of mucosa of transitional cell. Intertwining smooth muscle fibers called detrusor muscle that is not controlled by us and is involuntarily. The extracellular matrix is mainly composed of collagen located between mucosa and detrusor muscle and gives structural support to tissues. Normal bladder capacity is 400-600ml. Bladder muscles have elasticity and can be stretched to accommodate more urine inside.

The storage and emptying function of the bladder is essential for normal urinary tract function and continence of urine. The bladder accumulates urine at low pressure inside the bladder while the outlet is closed so there is no leakage (storage part, filling part). This part is abnormal in overactive bladder/urge incontinence.

During emptying, the bladder contracts in a regular and synchronized way, and the outlet opens so urine flows out. Normal frequency of micturition is usually 4-6 times per day, and urine that is voided is between 90 to 610 ml. Functional bladder capacity is usually 237 ml in the daytime and 379 ml at nighttime.

Parts of the Bladder Control System

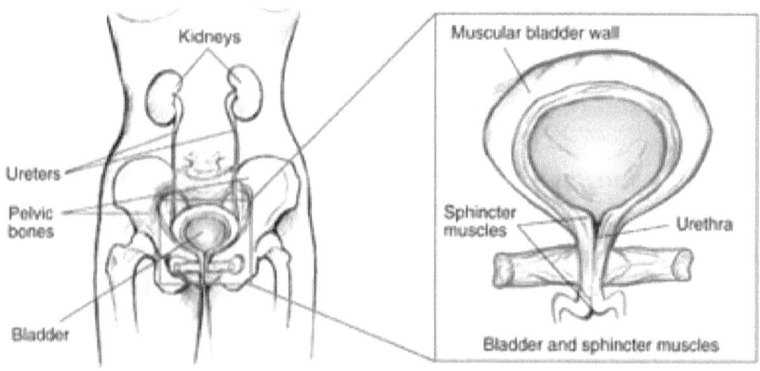

Front view, Bladder and sphincter muscles

Urethra

Urethra is a small muscular tube from the neck of the bladder to the front wall of the vagina in women or at the tip of the penis in men. The urethra is shorter (1-1.5 inches) in women than men (7-8 inches), and it is one of the reasons women have more frequent urinary tract infections than men do.

In the wall of urethra, there is a very competent group of muscles together called sphincters. Sphincters keep the urethra closed to prevent involuntary loss of urine (incontinence). In fact, there is no valvelike structure to function as a sphincter, but the urethra mainly acts as sphincter due to complex interaction between smooth and striated muscles.

The bladder neck that is at the junction of the urethra and bladder consists of involuntary smooth muscles also called internal sphincters. Striated muscles (voluntary muscles) around urethra are called external sphincter. The internal sphincter is involuntary; you cannot control it, and it is controlled by autonomic nervous system. You can control the external sphincter by relaxing it, and then you start urinating.

How Prevalent is Urinary Incontinence?

According to the World Health Organization, urinary incontinence affects approximately 200 million people worldwide. In the United States, between 13 to 33 million people have urinary incontinence. Because of a lack of a standardized definition of incontinence, these numbers vary. The sad finding is that less than 20% of people with incontinence receive medical attention and care.

The prevalence of urinary incontinence increases with age. It is about 10% of women at age thirty to 30% of women at age sixty-five. Men affected is about one-third compared to women until age eighty and after age eighty at the same rate as women.

The severity of incontinence increases with age as well, with 15-30% of women sixty-four and older living in nursing home communities having incontinence. In addition, more than 50% of all people in long-term care facilities suffer from incontinence.

The important issue is that more than half of people with incontinence do not report their incontinence problems to their doctors or even their families. The true prevalence may be much higher than these numbers.

Cost of Urinary Incontinence

The annual direct cost of urinary incontinence is estimated at more than $20 billion in a year. The total direct and indirect costs estimated are $6.3 billion or $3,600 per individual aged sixty-five and older.

Chapter Four

Am I at Risk?

Overview

The urinary tract organs, muscles, nerves, and the brain all work together to control the process of urination. The kidneys filter the blood to remove waste and water, producing urine. From the kidney, urine travels down tubes called ureters to the bladder. The bladder stores urine. Urine passes out of body by a tube called urethra. The sphincter is the functional, and not anatomical, valve that control flow of urine or stop it.

During normal urination, the brain sends signals to nerves in the spinal cord that causes the bladder to contract and force urine into the urethra. Nerves also send a message to the sphincter to relax so urine can pass. Urinary incontinence occurs if any of these organs do not function properly. Temporary urinary incontinence occurs usually secondary to urinary tract infection or irritants, vaginal infections, or some medications. Persistent urinary incontinence can occur as a result of damaged nerves, neurological disorders, pelvic muscle weakness, bladder activity, muscle overactivity, blockage of the urinary tract, and many other reasons.

Risk Factors

1. Lower Urinary Tract Condition

A. Affecting Both Sexes

i. Urinary Tract Infection

Infection of any part of your urinary tract can irritate and activate the sensory nerves and can cause incontinence. Urinary tract infection usually is accompanied by signs and symptoms of pain/discomfort/burning sensation while urinating (dysuria), foul-smelling urine, frequent urination (frequency), and a strong urge to urinate (urgency). A urinary tract infection is a common cause of incontinence. By treating the infection with antibiotics, incontinence would be cleared up.

ii. Obstruction

Obstruction can cause detrusor overactivity and urinary retention. We will discuss more specifics about causes of obstruction later.

iii. Bladder Abnormalities/Bladder Stones

Tumors, bladder stones, and interstitial cystitis can cause detrusoral abnormalities. If blood is present in the urine, talk to your doctor about further evaluations.

iv. Pelvic Surgery

Pelvic surgery, especially in women, increases the risk of urinary incontinence. At least 40% of women who have undergone a hysterectomy will develop urinary incontinence. In men, urinary incontinence can occur and persist after prostate cancer surgery.

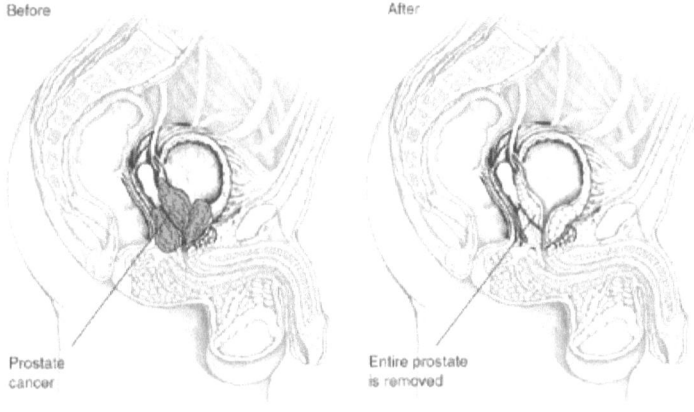

B. Affecting Women

i. Menopause and Loss of the Hormone Estrogen

There are estrogen receptors in your bladder, urethra, and pelvic muscles. Once a woman goes through menopause, hormone levels of estrogen are reduced, causing atrophy of tissues in the pelvic area.

After your periods end, your body stops making the female hormone estrogen. Estrogen controls how your body matures, your monthly periods, and body changes during pregnancy and breastfeeding. Estrogen may help keep the lining of the bladder and urethra healthy.

Lack of estrogen may contribute to weakness of bladder control muscles. Pressure from coughing, sneezing, or lifting can push urine through weakened muscles. This kind of leakage is called stress incontinence.

No study showed any benefit of taking estrogen for improving bladder control. In fact, one study showed worsening of bladder control after taking estrogens.

Estrogen changes will affect proper closure of the urethral sphincters. Bladder muscles become stiffer and less compliant so the bladder is not able to contract fully and is more prone to muscle spasm and urgency.

Estrogen reduction makes nerves in the bladder more sensitive and causes overactive bladder spasms and urgency. Decrease in blood estrogen level makes pelvic collagen fibers weaker and less effective in the urethra and pelvic structures.

ii. Pregnancy and Delivery

Half of women who were pregnant for the first time experience bladder control problems, especially in the last trimester. Pregnancy and childbirth sometimes cause stress incontinence.

Bladder control problems usually become worse with each additional pregnancy or with aging and hormonal changes. A forceful labor and episiotomy weakens the pelvic muscles and may cause nerve damage.

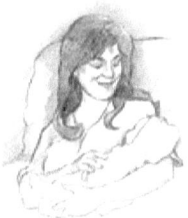

Pregnancy and childbirth sometimes cause stress incontinence

Nerves supplying pelvic muscles can be stretched or torn during delivery. Pudental nerves and pelvic nerves that are located on either side of birth canal can be damaged during delivery. Healthy nerves are essential for proper function of musculature and organs and maintenance of postpartum continence.

Sometimes forceps or vacuum suction used in delivery can damage pelvic musculature, nerves, and ligaments. Even large-sized babies can cause more injury that can lead to incontinence.

Hormonal fluctuation that is essential for delivering your baby can affect pelvic muscles. During breastfeeding, estrogen levels fall, causing pelvic muscle weakness and improper closure of the urethral sphincter.

Therefore, during breastfeeding, more episodes of incontinence occur. Even if you do not experience urinary or fecal incontinence following your delivery, some damage might have occurred. If you do not put an effort into strengthening your pelvic muscles, incontinence may be inevitable.

Any stress on the pelvic muscle may trigger the beginning of leakage. You do not want to set yourself up for future incontinence. Your next chest cold that makes you cough, your next pregnancy, or an increase in body weight can indicate how your pelvic muscles have weakened.

C. Affecting Men

Prostate Enlargement

Benign prostate enlargement or malignant lesions of the prostate can contribute to bladder muscle overactivity. In these situations, always talk to your doctor. Evaluation and treatment for possible prostate cancer is essential. Some medications (5a reductase) can reduce the size of prostate, and some (α blockers) may improve symptoms.

2.   Neurological Conditions

A. Neurological conditions affecting the brain: Alzheimer's disease, stroke, multi-infarct dementia, Parkinson's disease, and multiple sclerosis

These conditions affect the brain, so higher brain center control and inhibition over bladder is impaired. These neurological diseases can cause a range of different types of urinary incontinence. Most of them cause hyperactive bladder.

More than 80% of patients with multiple sclerosis have urinary dysfunction. They most commonly have urinary retention and may not be aware that their bladder is not completely emptied. They may feel urgency, nocturia, or incontinence. Multiple sclerosis causes involuntary bladder contractions that cause incontinence without awareness. In addition, overflow incontinence is common in multiple sclerosis.

With Parkinson's disease, urge incontinence and overflow incontinence coexist with an inability to go to the toilet in a timely manner because muscle rigidity contributes to incontinence. In addition, muscle weakness usually affects the sphincter muscles and causes fecal and urinary incontinence.

In Alzheimer's disease, the ability for self-care and self-hygiene diminishes. Locating a restroom may be a big problem for patients with incontinence. Incontinence incidents increase as the disease progresses.

B. Neurological conditions affecting the spinal cord: Cervical or lumbar stenosis (narrowing of the spine), disc herniation, spinal cord injury, multiple sclerosis

These conditions usually cause neurogenic overactive bladder and sometimes cause urinary retention. If urinary incontinence occurs because of these conditions, further evaluation is required. Talk to your doctor about it promptly.

C. Neurological conditions affecting peripheral nerves: Diabetic neuropathy, nerve injury

Diabetes mellitus causes neuropathy and urinary retention. In addition, poor blood glucose control (hyperglycemia) contributes to an increase in the amount of urine due to drawing water from your tissues (osmotic diuresis) and incident of incontinence. In addition, if you are diabetic, you are more susceptible to urinary infection and subsequent incontinence. Nerve injury especially in pelvic surgery causes low functional bladder capacity and urinary retention.

3. Systemic Conditions

A. Aging

Even normal aging can weaken your pelvic muscles, and your ability for holding urine decreases. It is a good idea to begin improving your muscle strength in the early stages or before you have a problem.

By aging, the bladder loses its elasticity so it cannot contract as before, and urine retention after urination is higher compared to younger people. By aging, the kidneys produce more urine during the night, and that causes more incontinence. Aging also causes overactivity of the bladder muscle. Decreased mobility seen in the elderly also contributes to incontinence. Prostate hypertrophy can cause incontinence in men after age forty.

B. Congestive Heart Failure

If your heart is weak and cannot pump blood properly, blood tends to pool to your legs while standing and sitting. This condition is called peripheral edema.

In the supine position, when you lie down for sleep, the blood in the legs and ankles goes back to the kidneys and more urine is produced during the night. This condition causes increased urinating during the night (nocturia). Volume overload because of congestive heart failure and diuretics that are used to treat this condition both cause increased urine production and incidents of incontinence. Proper timing of diuretics can make a big difference. Salt restriction, leg elevation, and support hose can be helpful.

C. Chronic cough

Chronic cough secondary to smoking or chronic lung diseases such as asthma or chronic obstructive pulmonary disease causes sudden increases in intra-abdominal pressure that can weaken your pelvic floor muscles. If you have lung problems or chronic cough, you should start exercising your pelvic muscles. The sooner you start exercises, the better the results you get.

D. Smoking

Smoking increases your risk of incontinence via the effect of nicotine on the bladder and increased detrusor muscle contractions. Smoking also causes incontinence through lung damage and chronic cough. This type of cough is usually harder and more frequent than a nonsmoker's cough.

E. Obesity

Obesity causes urinary incontinence by increasing intra-abdominal pressure and increased pressure over bladder and increased urethral mobility. In addition, obesity by impairing blood flow and nerves to the bladder and pelvic muscles promotes incontinence. Weight reduction can be a great help for obese men and women in controlling urinary incontinence.

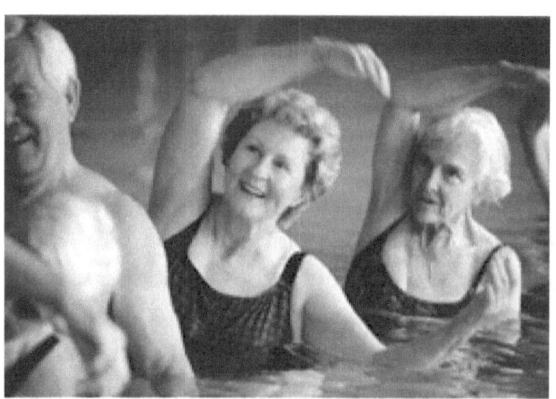

4.   Behavioral Conditions

A.   Restricted or Decreased Mobility

Impaired mobility that is usually associated with aging and chronic degenerative diseases can lead to incontinence in different ways. Restricted mobility hinders the speed and ability to self-toilet. Confinement to bed or using a wheelchair can place you at risk for developing incontinence.

Poor vision, arthritis, congestive heart failure, and medications side effects can decrease your movements. In addition, difficulty in unzipping your clothing in time may cause leakage. Sever osteoporosis and muscle weakness can contribute to incontinence. Treatment of underlying disorders, including physical therapy, is useful. Use of urinals, bedpans, and bedside commode are helpful.

B.   Certain Physical and Occupational Activity

There are some activities that increase pressure in the abdomen and thus increase downward pressure on the urinary bladder.

High impact exercises are more likely to produce symptoms of stress incontinence than low impact exercises. Sports causing increased pressure on bladder include basketball, volleyball, gymnastics, horseback riding, bodybuilding with heavy weights, and jumping.
Some occupations that involve heavy lifting increase risk of incontinence as well. Limited bathroom accessibility increases the risk too.

Lower impact activities and sports that have at least one foot touching the floor are low risk for incontinence. Examples are swimming, bicycling, walking, aerobics (low impact).

C.   Dehydration and Low Water Intake

If you do not drink adequate water in the fear of urinary loss incident, the produced urine would be very concentrated and would irritate bladder that causes more frequent urinating. In addition, concentrated urine can be an ideal environment for bacteria growth and urinary infection.

D. Excessive Intake of Caffeine or Alcohol

Excess alcohol and caffeine causes increase in urination and frequency of urination that can result in incontinence. Caffeine is found in coffee, tea, chocolate candies, soft drinks, many processed foods, as well as some of the over-the-counter medications like pain medications, allergy, stimulant, and some weight-loss drugs. Caffeine irritates your bladder, causing frequent urination that can increase the incident of incontinence.

E. Bowel Impaction and Constipation

If you are constipated, stool becomes hard and impacted. It can impose increased pressure over the bladder and cause incontinence. Enough hydration and suitable bowel regimen is very helpful.

5. Psychological Conditions

Chronic anxiety and learned voiding dysfunction can cause incontinence.

6. Medications

Some medications' side effects cause urinary dysfunction and incontinence.

Diuretic medications, especially the rapid acting ones, cause rapid increase in bladder volume, which precipitate urgency and bladder overactivity. Changing to a longer acting drug or adjusting the timing or dosage is beneficial.

Anticholinergic drugs, narcotics, calcium channel blockers (verapamil, nifedipine, diltiazem)—these drugs decrease bladder contractility and may cause urinary retention that leads to overflow incontinence.

Alpha-adrenergic drugs (doxazosin, perazosin)—these drugs are used for treatment of hypertension and benign prostate hypertrophy. In women, they cause stress incontinence and, in men, may lead to obstruction.

Antipsychotics drugs may impair mobility and response time

Chapter Five

Help! I Need Help

When experiencing incontinence, most people do not know what to do and how to get help. Some even think it is a normal part of aging or childbirth and delay seeking treatment. Unfortunately, both men and women delay seeking help. Women may wait more than three years to look for any professional help.

Before making any decisions, you should always consult with your physician. Today, there are many new ways to manage the problem of incontinence. If your doctor is reluctant to listen to you or treats this issue lightly, you may need to seek help from other doctors who have knowledge and experience in urinary incontinence. Having knowledge of treating incontinence nonsurgically, especially by behavioral therapy and biofeedback and nerve stimulation, are the skills you need to look for before deciding about incontinence surgery.

How to Find out the Cause of Urinary Incontinence

Report your symptoms, time of onset, duration, associated factors, and any possible pain to your doctor. It is better to write down what you would like to discuss with your doctor before your actual appointment.

Usually your doctor will ask most of the questions listed below. Read these and prepare your answers honestly and as accurately as possible.

- When did your incontinence start?
- Was your incontinence associated with a specific event like childbirth, surgery, menopause, or medical illness?

- How has incontinence changed overtime? Gotten better, worse, or remains the same?
- When do you lose urine? At night, during the day, or both?
- What time of day does incontinence occur?
- What relationship to activities does your incontinence have?
- What are your symptoms? Urgency, hesitancy, frequency, dysuria, episodes of leakage?
- What length of time has your problem with urinary incontinence existed?
- When was the onset of bladder dysfunction?
- Do you have urinary tract infection? Recent or chronically? How many times have you had urinary tract infection?
- What activities cause leakage? Is it associated with laughing, coughing, sneezing, or standing from sitting position?
- Do you leak urine while exercising?
- Have you lost urine during or after sex?
- Did urinary incontinence change your sexual habits?
- How frequently does leakage happen?
- How much urine do you lose during an accident? Teaspoon, tablespoon, half a cup, or more?
- What do you use to protect against leakage? A pad or diaper?
- How many times do you change your protection?
- Do you have an urge or warning before a bladder accident?
- How soon after warning does your bladder leakages occur?
- Do you lose urine while sitting still?
- Do you lose urine on the way to bathroom?
- How many times do you urinate during the day?
- How many times do you wake up to urinate at night?
- Do you wake up from sleep wet?
- How many glasses of water do you drink per day?
- How much caffeinated beverage do you drink during a day?
- Once on the toilet, how many minutes does it take to initiate urination?
- Describe the urinary stream when and how it starts once you try to initiate it.
- Is the stream continuous or on and off? How strong is the stream?
- Is there any pain with urination?
- Is there any straining needed to get urine out?

- Is there any postvoid dribbling?
- Do you feel you completely emptied your bladder?
- Did you ever notice any blood in your urine?
- Was there a change in odor or color of urine?
- Are you constipated or do you have abdominal bloating? Do you lose gas?
- Do you have any fecal incontinence?
- Do you have any history of any medical illness, for example, diabetes, congestive heart failure, arthritis, or kidney disease?
- Do you have any history of stroke, Parkinson's disease, or multiple sclerosis?
- Are you taking any medications? The complete list of medications including over-the-counter medications is needed.
- How many births did you have? How many vaginal deliveries did you have? Did you have episiotomy?
- Did you have any abdominal, pelvic, or back surgery?
- Did you have any urologic surgery before?
- Did you have any history of cancer or radiation therapy in your pelvic or abdominal area?
- Do you feel any protrusion from your vagina?
- In men, did you have any history of prostate enlargement or surgery?

What to Expect in a Physical Exam

You may need a complete physical exam that includes the following:

Abdominal Exam

The doctor would look for any

- mass/organ enlargement;
- pain, discomfort, fullness;
- ascites or fluid in the abdomen;
- surgical incisions.

He would listen to bowel sounds and would pay attention to hypo-activity or overactivity of bowel sounds.

Pelvic and Genital Exam in Women

During this exam, the doctor would evaluate the following:

- Dryness/redness/thinning on mucosa (suggestive of atrophic vaginitis)
- Your skin in the perineal area
- Measure your vaginal PH (A vaginal PH of more than 7 is correlated to atrophic symptoms and hypoestrogenism. In these cases, use of topical estrogen may be helpful.)
- Your pelvic muscle strength
- Any structural abnormalities like uterine prolapse
- Uterine fibroids

Genitalia Exam in Men

Doctor usually does a complete exam of the penis, scrotum, testes, foreskin, and glands.

Rectal Exam

During a rectal exam in women the doctor will be assessing

- your rectal sphincter tone;
- your prostate size;
- your pelvic muscle strength;
- fecal impaction.

In men, doctor would assess the following:

- Your sphincter tone
- Size, symmetry and texture of prostate
- Any mass
- Fecal impaction
- Your pelvic floor muscle strength

Neurological Exam

This type of exam assesses your ability to comprehend your condition and situation. It should address the following:

- Your short- and long-term memory
- Your moods
- Speech patterns
- Your ability to perform fine movement tasks
- How you interpret the sensation of urination
- Your reflexes
- Difficulty walking or getting around
- Specific diseases like multiple sclerosis, Parkinson's disease or Alzheimer's disease
- Any deficit caused by a past condition such as a stroke

Assessment of Your Functions and Ability

The doctor will want to assess your ability to move around.

- Can you get to a bathroom on time by yourself ?
- Do you need a little assistance for going to bathroom?
- Do you need a wheelchair, walker, or cane to get to toileting facilities?
- Do you take any drugs that would restrict you from getting to the bathroom on time?
- Does anything else keep you from getting to the bathroom?
- Are the bathrooms handicap assessable?
- Are there any job-related limitations that are making it difficult for you to reach the toilet on time?
- Can you undress (unbutton or unzip) in time to use the toilet.

Assessment of Environmental Barriers

- Are toileting aids such as bedside commodes or urinals available at the bedside?
- Can you rise from your furniture easily? (Is furniture height more than 19 inches?)
- Do you know where the bathroom is?
- Is it easy to go to the bathroom?
- Is there adequate light to go to the bathroom during the night?
- Do you use stairs to reach to bathroom?
- Are bathrooms wheelchair and walker accessible?
- Is there enough light and color contrast in the bathroom?

- Can you easily unbutton or unzip your clothing?
- Are toilet seats at least 17 inches in height so that you can sit and rise comfortably?
- Are grab bars available in the bathroom and within your reach?

Bladder and Bowel Diary

Bladder diary is a record of fluid intake and trips to the bathroom. The bladder diary will help your doctor determine patterns and frequency of urination during the day and night. It also will help you to keep track of your urinary patterns. Using your bladder diary will identify triggers (like certain foods or beverages) that you otherwise might not be aware.
A minimal of three days is required to get a good idea of your situation. Your chart should include

- Time
- Foods
- Fluids
- Did you urinate?
- Other circumstances?
- What kind/how much?
- How many times/much leakage? Urge to urinate?
- What were you doing?
- How many pads do you use each day?
- Type of pads

Useful Tests

Urinalysis

Urinalysis is a test to determine if any red blood cells, leukocytes (white blood cells), bacteria, and glucose are present in the urine sample.

Bacteria in the urine sample (bacturia) do not always need antibiotic treatment. Red blood cells in your urine samples (hematuria) are a serious issue and needs the attention of a physician.

If you have urinary tract infection, treat it before starting therapy for incontinence.

Postvoid Residual Urine Test

This test assesses residual urine volume within 15 to 20 minutes after a person uses the toilet. When you have finished urinating, you may still have some urine usually 1 or 2 ounces remaining in the bladder. To measure this postvoid residual, the doctor or the nurse may remove the remaining urine by catheter (a thin tube that can be gently glided into urethra). Ultrasound equipment that send harmless sound waves to the bladder for creating a picture of the bladder can also be used and is safer and easier.
Residual volume of less than 50 ml is normal and more than 200 ml is not normal and is a sign of a problem. It may mean there is an obstruction or your bladder contractions are impaired.

People at risk of having high residual volume are the following:

- Older patients
- Men, especially those with history of enlarged prostate
- Diabetes mellitus patients
- History of a neurological disorder
- Those who take anticholinergics medications (that interfere with bladder emptying)
- Those having suprapubic tenderness or distention
- Those with recurrent urinary tract infection

Pad Test

A pad test is very simple test to determine the amount of urine leakage you experience during a routine day. This determination is done by weighing the pads.

How Do I Perform the Test?

Your doctor will give you a number of absorbent pads and plastic bags of standard weigh. You are told to wear the pad for 1-2 hours and then seal it in a bag. Your doctor's office personnel then weigh the bags to see how much urine has been caught in the pad. Usually twenty-four hours is enough for assessing the amount of leakage.

Ultrasound

Transrectal Ultrasound

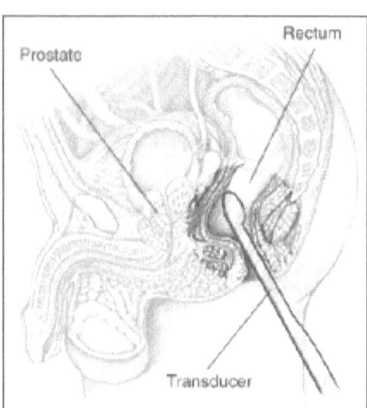

Transrectal ultrasound

For an ultrasound, or sonography, a technician holds a device called a transducer that sends harmless sound waves into the body and catches them as they bounce back off the organs inside to create a picture on a monitor. In abdominal ultrasound, the technician slides the transducer over the surface of your abdomen for images of the bladder and kidneys. In transrectal ultrasound, the technician uses a wand inserted in the rectum for images of the prostate.

Urodynamic Test

Urodynamic testing is a special test that evaluates the bladder's ability to store urine and empty steadily and completely. It also assesses flow of urine as it leaves the bladder and goes through the urethra

Urodynamic study can help to establish correct diagnosis during the initial workup and measurement of your improvement or deterioration. Sometimes this test is ordered prior to urinary tract or pelvic floor surgery.

How Should I Prepare?

You should drink enough fluids to have a full bladder before the test. Your doctor may instruct you to skip some medicines or foods.

Uroflowmetry

Uroflowmeter Equipment

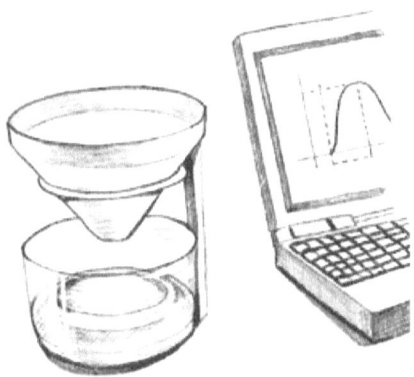

Uroflowmeter equipment

Uroflowmetry is the measurement of urine speed and volume. A uroflowmeter measures the amount of urine and flow rate (how fast the urine comes out). The doctor may ask you to urinate privately into a toilet that contains a collection device and a scale. This equipment creates a graph that shows changes in flow rate from second to second. Your doctor can see peak flow rate and the time it takes to get there. If your bladder muscle is weak or urine flow is obstructed, the result of the test would be abnormal

Cystometry

Cystometry is measurement of bladder pressure. A cystometrogram (CMG) measures how much your bladder can hold, how much pressure builds up inside your bladder as it stores urine, and how full it is when you feel the urge to urinate. The doctor will use a catheter to empty your bladder completely. Then a special, smaller catheter with a pressure-measuring tube will be used to fill you slowly with warm water. Another catheter may be placed in the rectum to record pressure there as well. The doctor would ask you how your bladder feels and when you feel the need to urinate. The volume of water and bladder pressure will be recorded. The doctor may ask you to cough or strain during procedure. The doctor can identify involuntary bladder contractions.

Measurement of Leak Point Pressure

While your bladder is being filled for CMG, it may suddenly contract and squeeze some water out without warning. The cystometer will record the pressure at the point when the leakage occurred. This reading would give information about the kind of bladder problem you have. The doctor may ask you to exhale while holding your nose and mouth to apply abdominal pressure to the bladder or cough or shift positions. These actions help your doctor to evaluate your sphincter muscle.

Pressure Flow Study

After CMG, the doctor would ask you to empty your bladder so that the catheter can measure the pressure required to urinate. This pressure flow study helps to identify bladder outlet obstruction that men may experience with prostate enlargement. Bladder outlet obstruction in women can occur with a fallen bladder or after pelvic surgery.

Electromyography

If your doctor suspects nerve damage, he/she may use electromyography. This test measures the muscle activity in urethra and rectum. Muscle activity is recorded on a machine and the patterns would show whether urethra and bladder are coordinated.

After the Test

You may have mild discomfort for a few hours after these tests. Drinking 2-3 glasses of water each hour for 2 hours would help. A warm damp washcloth over urethral opening can help.

Your doctor may give you antibiotic for up to 2 days to prevent an infection. Inform your physician if you develop fever, flank pain, see blood clots, or have difficulty urinating.

Chapter Six

Treatment of Urinary Incontinence

Appropriate treatment of urinary incontinence depends on the accurate diagnosis of the underlying etiology.

Urge Incontinence

Patients with isolated urge incontinence (detrusor instability) are best treated with conservative treatment options including bladder retraining, behavioral modification, biofeedback, functional electrical stimulation, and pharmacologic therapy.

Stress Incontinence

- Patients with isolated genuine stress incontinence, because of urethral hypermobility or intrinsic sphincter deficiency, may be candidates for conservative therapy including Kegel exercises, pelvic muscle rehabilitation with biofeedback, electrical stimulation, or medications.
- An initial course of conservative therapy is recommended for all patients with follow-up assessment in 2 to 3 months.
- Surgery should be considered for patients with persistent urinary leakage or those who desire surgical correction.

Mixed Incontinence

Patients with mixed incontinence should be initially offered a trial of conservative treatment consisting of Kegel exercises, bladder training, behavioral therapy, pelvic muscle rehabilitation, biofeedback, nerve stimulation, and if they do not improve, medications. Surgery usually is reserved for those who did not show improvement with a conservative treatment and who are willing to have surgery.

Secondary Causes of Incontinence

Patients with secondary causes of incontinence should be treated on an individual basis.

Behavioral Modification

1. Dietary Restriction and Modification

Avoid alcohol. Alcohol is an irritant to the bladder and can cause incontinence and frequent urination.

Avoid spicy foods. Highly spiced foods can cause bladder irritation.

Avoid red food dye. Red food dye is found in many processed meats, hot dogs, sausages, and baked goods. It may irritate the bladder lining and causes worsening of incontinence.

Avoid sugar and artificial sweetener. Avoid consuming high quantities of sugars. These have irritant effect on the bladder.

Avoid large amounts of citrus fruits. Large amount consumption of citrus fruits can irritate the bladder.

Drink adequate water. Drinking too much fluid at one time can overwhelm the bladder. The best strategy is to spread water during the day. Also avoid drinking lots of water after dinner to prevent nighttime frequent voiding.

On the other hand, dehydration and concentrated urine is an irritant to the bladder. In addition, inadequate water intake causes constipation and can further worsen your incontinence problem. A healthy adult usually drinks about eight 8-ounce cups of water per day.

2. Quit smoking

Nicotine in cigarette is an irritant to bladder mucosa. Coughing, associated with smoking, causes increase in leakage. In addition, chronic cough can weaken your pelvic muscles.

3. Lose weight if you are overweight.

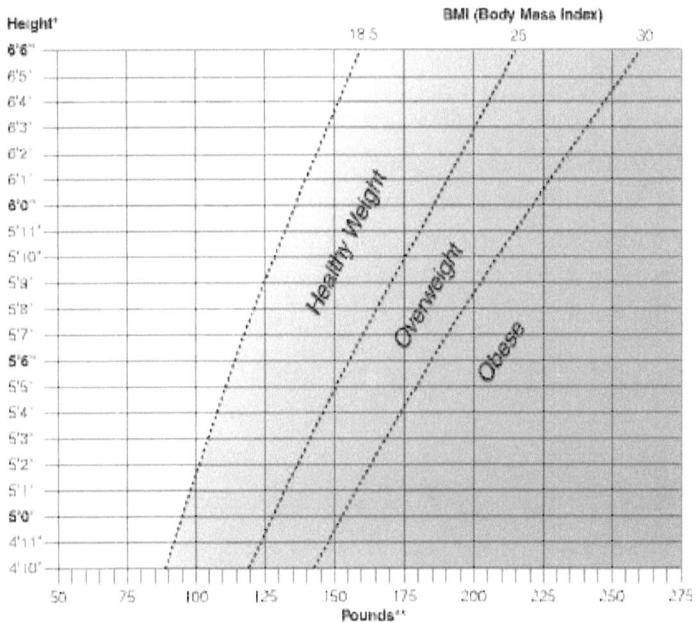

Being overweight can lead to a number of health problems, so losing your extra weight can help with a variety of concerns. These extra pounds also can cause and worsen incontinence symptoms. Weight loss, even moderate (up to 5% of body weight), can help with your incontinence symptoms. Extra pounds can cause pressure on the intra-abdominal organs and increase the episodes and symptoms of incontinence.

Bladder Retraining: Is It Helpful for Me?

Bladder retraining is the mainstay of treatment for urge and mixed incontinence and is effective in reducing episodes of stress incontinence. Bladder retraining helps the bladder to hold urine for longer periods.

People using bladder retraining should have

- intact cognition;
- recognize sensation of urge;
- ability to follow structured programs.

What Is It?

Bladder retraining is simply timed voiding. It helps to distend the bladder progressively and allows you to regain critical control over voiding pattern. You teach your bladder new habits.

You are instructed to empty your bladder at preassigned times during the waking hours. By reviewing your voiding diary, your current voiding interval is estimated. At first week, your time between your bathroom trips is set at less than your current interval, and then it is gradually increased over an eight-week period usually half an hour per week.

How to Suppress the Urge to Urinate

- When the urge starts, do not rush to the bathroom. Stay calm.
- When the urge grows, squeeze your pelvic muscles 5-6 times quickly.
- When the urge sensation peaks, take slow deep breaths and wait until the urge subsides. Try to distract yourself or repeat self-encouraging statements.
- When the urge stops, wait few more minutes. If you can, wait until your scheduled time. Walk slowly to the bathroom. Do not run to the bathroom as running increases the bladder's contraction that increases the incontinence incident.
- Keep an accurate bladder diary. Your doctor can decide when to change your interval by reviewing your diary. Usually if you can go 2 days without an episode of urinary incontinence, the interval increased by 30-60 minutes.

Pelvic Muscle Rehabilitation

Pelvic muscle rehabilitation can reduce the severity of incontinent episodes by strengthening the pelvic muscles and reestablishing support to the bladder neck. It also strengthens the muscular component of urethral closure mechanism using principles of strength training.

Pelvic muscle rehabilitation is very useful in stress urinary incontinence in women with poor pelvic support and in men after prostate surgery. In addition, it is useful in patients with urge or mixed incontinence. Unfortunately, after verbal instruction, less than 30% of women can perform pelvic muscle exercises correctly. Pelvic floor exercises can be enhanced using biofeedback with intravaginal pressure probes or perineal electrodes.

Instruction to interrupt urination on a regular basis is not physiologic and sometimes dangerous and is doomed to fail.

The recommended regimen is the following:

- Three sets of 8-12 slow velocity contractions. You need to sustain these contractions for 6-8 seconds each.
- You need to perform these exercises 3-4 times a week.
- You should continue these exercises at least 15-20 weeks and preferably lifelong. Like any exercise, they are effective as long as you continue doing them.

Please refer to chapter 6 about details of pelvic muscle exercises. Please watch the accompanying DVD carefully.

Cognitively Impaired Patients

Behavioral methods can be used for cognitively impaired individuals as well. These methods include the following:

- Habit training (timed voiding with intervals based upon individual's usual voiding schedule as is determined by voiding dairy)
- Scheduled voiding (timed voiding using a logical set interval like every 2-3 hours)
- Prompt voiding.
  1. Patients encourage reporting their continence status.
  2. Patients prompted to toilet on a scheduled basis
  3. Positive feedback when patient is continent.

Biofeedback Therapy

What is Biofeedback?

Biofeedback therapy is simply learning your body's responses. Biofeedback is a system that uses monitoring procedures that give you feedback on body-specific physiologic responses like muscle activity, heart rate, skin temperature, and brain electrical activity. It gives greater awareness of the internal process from enhanced sensory information.

There are different kinds of biofeedback including EEG, EMG, electrodermal, respiration, heart rate, blood-pulse volume, and heart-rate variability. In biofeedback therapy, the patient learns how to control their internal biology. Therapists serve as a coach offering suggestions tailored to the individual.

Biofeedback in Urinary Incontinence

Many people have difficulty in isolating muscles they need to contract in order to exercise and strengthen the pelvic muscles. Using biofeedback can be of great help, and you can learn how to contract these muscles properly.

Biofeedback can monitor electrical activity of pelvic floor muscles The goal of using biofeedback in the treatment of urinary incontinence is to alter the responses of detrusor and pelvic muscles, which control urine loss. You also would learn how to control the external sphincter.

Biofeedback therapy is not only helpful for treatment of muscle dysfunction, but it also helps you locate the pelvic muscles. It increases your awareness of muscle tension using electrical or pressure devices. By changing the graph or light when correct muscles resqueezed or tightened, you would know if you are using the correct muscles.

An EMG probe or surface electrodes measure electrical signals from the sphincter muscle. The information about status and condition of pelvic muscles is then stored and processed. This allows you to see them in the form of lights, images, or sounds.

Biofeedback can be done sitting, standing, or lying down. In a typical session, you may use an intravaginal or a perineal electrode (over the skin adjacent to pelvic muscle in perineum).

The therapist would ask you to contract the pelvic muscles. Your muscle contraction, strength, and pattern are registered and compared to ideal contractions. You would learn how to change your contractions to be as close as possible to the ideal contractions. You would learn how to selectively contract and relax these muscles while you keep abdominal muscles relaxed. In addition, you would learn how to respond to urge sensation. Behavioral methods are more effective than medications. In one trial, behavioral therapy with biofeedback reduced incontinence accidents by 81% compared to 69% reduction by drug therapy.

Home Biofeedback

You may need more exercises with help of biofeedback at home. To assist practicing pelvic muscles at home, your doctor may prescribe portable biofeedback units. These units usually record your progression.

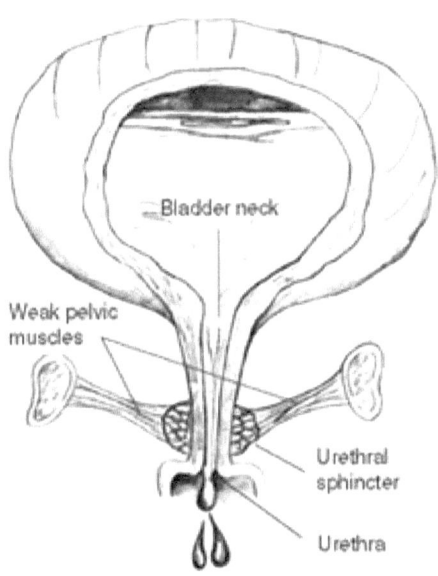

Front view of bladder. Weak pelvic muscles allow urine leakage.

Electrical Stimulation

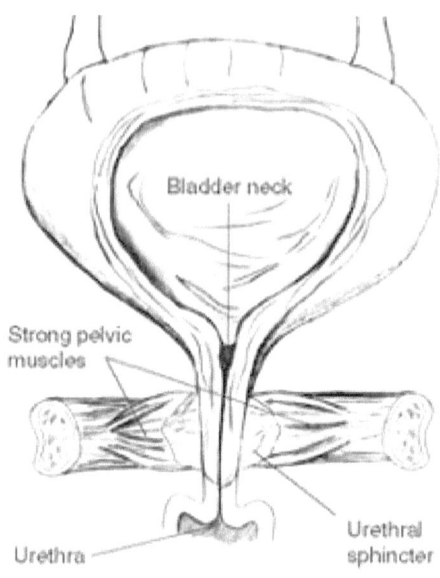

Front view of bladder, Weak pelvic muscles allow urine leakage.
Strong pelvic muscles keep the urethra closed.

Electrical stimulation is effective in the treatment of stress, urge, and mixed incontinence. This treatment modality is helpful in patients who is unable to properly perform pelvic muscle exercises or in patients whose levator muscle cannot contract effectively.

The best and practical regimen is electrical stimulation at frequency of 10-50 hertz for 20 minutes once or twice daily.

The stimulation should be at the maximum intensity patient can tolerate without pain. After 8-12 weeks of treatment usually 52-77% improvement is seen. The therapeutic benefits of nerve stimulation extend more than the actual period of stimulation therapy. In one study, benefits were present after two years of active treatment.

Pelvic floor electrical stimulation is very beneficial for men and women who are unable to contract these muscles on command. Pelvic muscle stimulation contracts the pelvic muscles for you. The equipment delivers an electrical stimulation through an intravaginal or intra-anal small tube (electrode) or skin electrodes on perineal area. The procedure is usually performed in your doctor's office.

This signal causes muscles to contract. The stimulation is not painful; it feels like a vibration in the muscle. Electrical stimulation is usually combined with pelvic floor exercise program.

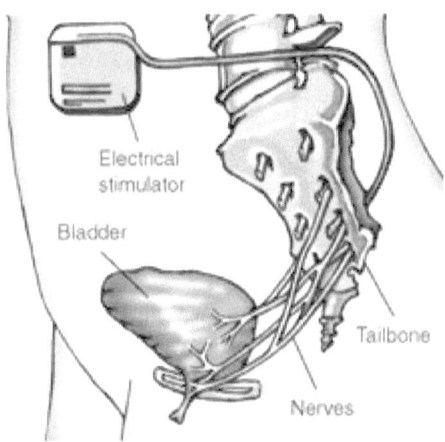

Vaginal Weights and Cones

Vaginal cones help you to isolate and strengthen pelvic muscles. The cones are made of plastics and look like smooth white suppositories. They are in identical size and shape but of increasing weight, from less than an ounce to few ounces. You insert the cone into the vagina (like a tampon) and then grip your pelvic muscles tightly to prevent them from falling. Ten minutes 2 times a day is usually a good start for strengthening your muscles. After the exercises, remove the cones and wash them with soap and water. Increase the cones' weight gradually. You may also practice holding cones and weights while jumping, laughing, and coughing. Do not use them if you have an infection or during menstruation.

Extracorporeal Magnetic Innervation (EXMI) Technology

This technology helps you to exercise your pelvic muscles without active participation in the exercises.

During treatment, you sit fully clothed in a special chair that has extracorporeal magnetic innervation EXMI technology embedded in the seat.

The seat produces highly focused pulsed magnetic fields. Pelvic floor muscles contract and relax with each magnetic pulse. No active participation is required from patients. The EXMI technology does the exercise for the patient.

Treatments are painless and are usually 20 minutes, and it is recommended for 8 weeks twice a week. If you have metal prosthesis or metal intrauterine devices (IUD), you're recommended not to use this technology.

Chapter Seven

Medications

Based on your history and physical examination and diagnostic evaluations, medications can be prescribed to control urinary incontinence.

Urge Incontinence/Overactive Bladder

1. Anticholinergics

These drugs block the nerve signals that cause frequent urination and urgency. These drugs relax muscles and prevent bladder spasms and can prevent urgency or urgency incontinence. They can be used until biofeedback or bladder training helps control the problem.

Some of these oral medications are the following:

- Oxybutynin (Ditropan)
- Tolterodine (Detrol)
- Trospium chloride (Sanctura)
- Enablex (Darifenacin)
- Vesicare (Solifenacin succinate)

Most common side effects of these medications are the following:

1. Dry mouth
2. Blurred vision
3. Dry skin
4. Rapid heart rate
5. Constipation
6. Confusion

7. Headache
8. Flushing
9. Drowsiness
10. Urinary retention

If you take medicine to treat an overactive bladder, you should take several precautions.

- Wear sunglasses if your eyes become more sensitive to light.
- Take care not to become overheated.
- Chew gum or suck on sugarless hard candy to avoid dry mouth.

Different medicines can affect the nerves and muscles of the urinary tract in different ways. Pills to treat edema and swelling or high blood pressure (diuretics) may increase your urine output and contribute to bladder control problems. Talking to your doctor about may be changing one of the medications you are taking now can solve the problem without adding another medication.

2. Imipramine

Imipramine belongs to a group of medications called tricyclic antidepressant. Impramine has both anticholinergics and alpha adrenergic effects. These drugs relax bladder muscles and tighten urethral muscles. In high doses, they are used for depression; in low doses, they are used for treating urinary incontinence. These medications can be helpful in bladder filling and urine storage. They can be used instead or in combination of anticholinergics. Imipramine has serious side effects. Some of the possible side effects are the following:

1. Dry mouth
2. Blurred vision
3. Urinary retention
4. Constipation
5. Sedation and drowsiness
6. Weight gain
7. Rapid heart rate

Stress Incontinence

This type of incontinence occurs when muscles around the urethra do not sufficiently close, especially when you cough or sneeze. There is no approved drug for stress incontinence.

Mixed Incontinence

Mixed incontinence is a combination of urgency incontinence and stress incontinence. This occurs when the bladder wall has spasms, and the sphincter muscles are weak and cannot prevent leaking. Anticholinergics drug might be helpful.

Treatment of Urinary Incontinence by Medication in Men

Medicines can affect bladder control in different ways. Some medicines help prevent incontinence by blocking abnormal nerve signals that make the bladder contract at the wrong time. Others slow production of urine. Some medications relax the bladder or shrink the prostate. Before prescribing a new medicine, may be changing one of the drugs you already take is beneficial.

Your doctor may choose one of the following groups of medicines.

- *Alpha blockers.* These medications are used to treat problems caused by enlarged prostate and bladder outlet obstruction. They relax the smooth muscle of the prostate and bladder neck. They allow normal urine flow and prevent abnormal bladder contractions that cause urge incontinence.

  Examples are terazosin (Hytrin), doxazosin (Cardura), and tamsulosin (Flomax).

- *Antispasmotics.* These drugs relax the bladder muscles and relieve spasms. Examples are propantheline (Pro-Banthine), tolerodine (Detrol LA), and oxybutynin (Ditropan XL).

  They have side effects like dry mouth, blurred vision, and headache and flushing; you may need to take precautions as described with anticholinergics in previous pages.

- *5-alpha reductase inhibitor.* These medications inhibit production of male hormone DHT, which is responsible for prostate enlargement. These drugs shrink prostate size and relieve voiding problems.

  Examples are finasteride (Proscar) and dutasteride (Avodart).

- *Imipramine (Tofranil).* This drug belongs to tricyclic antidepressants; these medicines relax muscles and block nerve signals that cause bladder spasm. It is used in children bedwetting as well.

Caution

If you have glaucoma, most of these medications can be dangerous for you. Consult your physician before taking any medications.

Chapter Eight

Prosthetic Devices: Inserts and Plugs for Managing Urinary Incontinence

Nonsurgical Methods for Bladder Support in Women

Intravaginal Devices and Pessaries

Introl

This is a ring-shaped polythene object with two prongs pointing superiorly. It is placed inside the vagina. The prongs fit under the urethra and holds it up. It supports the bladder neck, keeps the urethra from moving, and prevents leaking.

Introl is useful if you have incontinence during stressful physical activity such as jogging, jumping, or aerobics. It comes in different sizes. You may remove it after activity, wash it with water, and keep it for the next time you need it.

Pessary

Pessary is a plastic device that fits into the vagina to help support the uterus, vagina, and bladder or rectum.

Pessary is helpful for prolapse, cystocele, or rectoele. It is helpful in stress urinary incontinence.

There are many types of pessary available, and usually after few trials, you and your doctor may find the right size and type. It may cause vaginal irritation and increase in vaginal discharge.

You need to notify your doctor promptly if you have problems with urinating or bowel movement or if you have pain.

Implants/Bulking Agents

Urethral injections. Adding bulk to the tissue around the bladder opening helps keep the urethra closed.

Implants. Implants are substances injected into tissues around the urethra. The implants add bulk and help to close the urethra to reduce stress incontinence. Different materials have been used. Collagen (a fibrous natural tissue from cows) and fat from the patient's body are more popular. Your doctor under local anesthesia can inject implants.

One of the disadvantages of collagen is that the body slowly eliminates it. So injections must be repeated after a certain time. Before collagen injection, your doctor would do a skin test to make sure you are not allergic to collagen.

Extraurethral Devices

Occlusive devices.

Continence control pad. These are soft adhesive rubber pad. These patches fit over urethra opening, block the flow of urine and prevent leakage. Patches can be used for few hours and it is ideal for incontinence during exercise.

Chapter Nine

Surgery

Doctors usually suggest surgery to alleviate incontinence only after other treatments have been tried without success. In this book, we are discussing about a few procedures that are more common. There are many other procedures that are not mentioned in this book, and you may discuss it with your doctor.

Surgery for Incontinence in Women

The goal of surgery for incontinence treatment in women is restoring the bladder and the urethra to their normal position. Common surgery for stress incontinence involves pulling the bladder up to a more normal position.

Bladder Neck Suspension

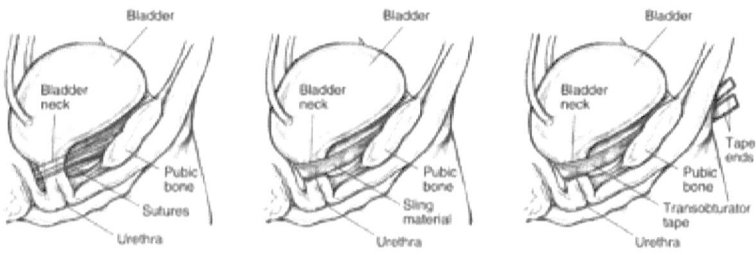

Working through an incision in the vagina or abdomen, the surgeon raises the bladder and secures it with a string attached to a muscle, ligament, or bone. Therefore, the bladder and the urethra are then pulled back to the normal position.

Sling Procedure

For several cases of stress incontinence, surgeons may secure the bladder with a wide sling. This procedure holds up the bladder and compresses the bottom of the bladder and the top of the urethra, preventing leakage.

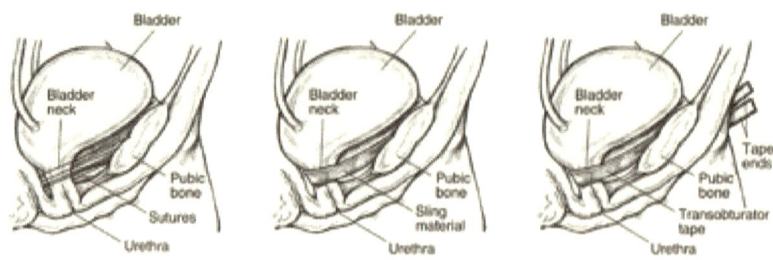

Sling in place, secured to the pubic bone

Artificial Urinary Sphincter in Women

Artificial urinary sphincter in women have three parts: a cuff that that goes around urethra, a pump that goes in the labia, and a reservoir that is in the abdomen. When you want to urinate, you press the pump. The side effects are mechanical failure, infection, or erosion of the sphincter.

Surgery in Men

Implantation of an Artificial Urinary Sphincter

Some men may eliminate urine leakage with an artificial sphincter, an implanted device that keeps the urethra closed until you are ready to urinate. It does not solve incontinence caused by uncontrolled bladder contractions. This device helps people who have incontinence because of weak sphincter muscles or because of nerve damage that interferes with sphincter muscle function.

This device has three parts: a cuff that fits around the urethra, a small balloon reservoir placed in the abdomen, and pump placed in the scrotum. The cuff is filled with liquid that makes it fit tightly around the urethra to prevent urine from leaking. By pressing the pump with your fingers, you can cause the cuff to deflate. This removes pressure from the urethra allowing urine from the bladder to pass. When your bladder is empty, the cuff automatically refills in the next three to five minutes and keeps the urethra tightly closed.

Male Sling Procedure

In a sling procedure, the surgeon creates a support for the urethra by wrapping a strip of material around the urethra and attaching the ends of the strip to the pelvic bone. The sling keeps constant pressure on the urethra so that it does not open until the patient consciously releases the urine.

Chapter Ten

Natural Cures for Urinary Incontinence

Use of herbs in treating urinary incontinence and urinary problems has a long history, may be as long as the history of human life. Some of the herbal medicines that are used include the following:

Butterbur

This plant was used to treat the plague during the Middle Ages. This plant is a natural painkiller and is usually nonaddictive. Butterbur's active ingredient is called petasin. This compound decreases the spasm in many muscles and blood vessels, including bladder muscle. It may be helpful for migraine headache.

There are some reports that some ingredients in butterbur can cause cancer. More studies are needed to determine the risks and benefits of this herb.

To Improve Incontinence by Improving Nerve Function or To Improve Nerve Function

Ginkgo

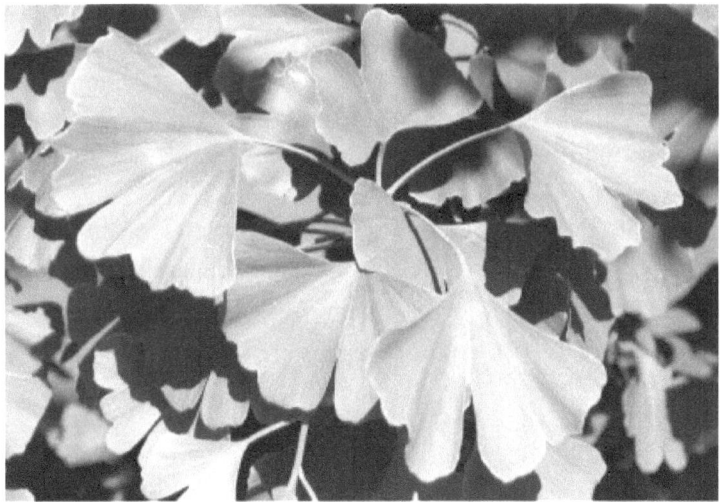

Ginkgo leaf extracts have a wide range of biological activities. It improves short-term memory, has a protective effect on the blood-brain barrier, and an antiradical (antioxidant) effect. It increases vasodilation and peripheral blood flow rate in capillary vessels and end arteries.

Gingko can help to regenerate nerves and help to relax smooth muscles. It can be helpful in incontinence caused by nerve dysfunction.

Herbs That Improve Incontinence by Prevention of Urinary Tract Infections

Cranberry

Urinary tract infections are serious health problems affecting millions of people. Each year, urinary tract infections account for about 10 million doctor visits. Most infections arise from one type of bacteria, *Escherichia coli*, which normally live in the colon.

Usually, the latest infection stems from a strain or type of bacteria that is different from the infection before it, indicating a separate infection. The ability of bacteria to attach to cells lining the urinary tract is an important factor.

Cranberry Use

Traditionally, urinary tract infections are treated with antibiotics, but these are expensive, can have side effects, and may lead to resistance.

Therefore, physicians suggest additional steps that patients can take on their own to avoid infection, including drinking cranberry juice.

Although cranberry juice is the form of cranberries most widely used, other cranberry products include cranberry powder in hard or soft gelatin capsules.

Mechanism of Action

Current belief is that the prevention of urinary tract infections is achieved by inhibiting the infecting bacteria, E. coli, from adhering to uroepithelial cells. Bacterial adherence to these cells is a critical step in the development of infection. Cranberry juice acts by preventing adhesion. Thus, the causative bacteria are washed away, preventing their colonization of the urinary tract.

Safety

Cranberry taken orally in food amounts appears safe although ingesting large amounts may result in diarrhea and other gastrointestinal symptoms. Safety of amounts greater than that consumed in foods is unknown.

Corn Silk

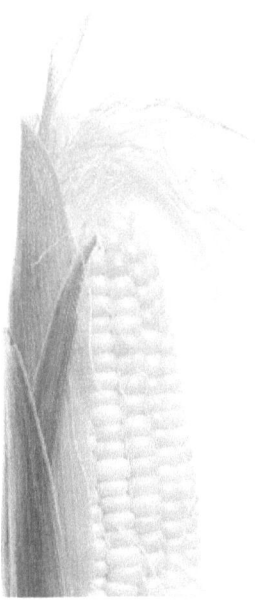

A North American native plant first grown by farmers in Mexico, corn (*Zea mays*) has been harvested for over 7,000 years. The genus name *Zea* means "cause of life," and the species name *mays* means "mother."

Corn silk is the soft fine silky yellowish hairlike threads that stick out of the corn ear. Corn silk has a long history of healing and also use in cosmetics. Corn silk is used to treat bladder infections, kidney stones, infections of the prostate gland, and urinary tract infections. It is also used as a diuretic and anti-inflammatory. Corn silk reduces painful symptoms and swelling due to inflammatory process and bladder infections. It is used for support of urinary system.

Safety: More research is needed to determine its safety.

Goldenseal

For many years and generations, goldenseal has been used by Native Americans. It is known for its antimicrobial and anti-inflammatory effect.

Goldenseal contains berberine, an alkaloid that may prevent urinary tract infections by preventing bacteria from adhering to the wall of the urinary bladder. Goldenseal may help in the treatment of urinary tract infections. Safety of this herb is not determined. Do not use it if pregnant or nursing. More research needed for determination of safety of this herb. It can be used as tea or capsules.

Uva Ursi

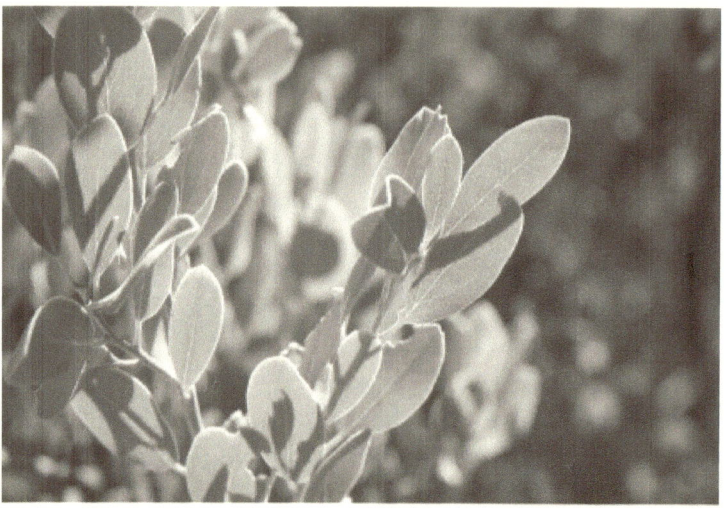

Uva ursi is a plant also known as bearberry. The leaves, not the berries, contain active ingredients. The most important ingredient is arbutin, which has antibacterial activity. Uva ursi is used in herbal medicinal teas to disinfect the urine. It may also act as a mild diuretic. It is also effective in treatment of cystitis and kidney stones. Arbutin is absorbed via the gastrointestinal tract and excreted via urine. In alkaline urine, it is active and has septic effect on urinary tract. Do not take if you are pregnant or lactating. Treatments should not be more than seven days.

More research needed for determination of safety of this herb.

Herbs That Improving Incontinence Caused by Renal Stones

Couch Grass

This herb has a long folk history of treating kidney and bladder stones. In folk medicine, it has been used for gout, bladder infections, urinary stones, chronic skin problems, and constipation. Its effectiveness for these problems has not been scientifically verified. The rhizome, root, and seeds are all used for medicinal purposes.

Couch grass is a natural diuretic (draws water from the body). It can wash out the urinary tract during infections. It can also destroy or inhibit the growth of bacteria and molds. It is recommended for prostitis, cystitis, and urethritis (urinary tract inflammations). It assists the body in eliminating stones from kidney and urinary bladder. Its high mucilage content makes it useful as a cough remedy.

Although couch grass is usually considered a troublesome weed, it has been used for centuries for medical purposes. It can be used as a tea or extract.

Safety is not determined, and more research is needed for safety information of this herb. Do not take it if you are pregnant or nursing. In some people, it can cause electrolyte imbalance.

Hydrangea, a natural diuretic helpful in treating kidney and bladder stones, is one of the most powerful solvents of stones. It both helps with the expulsion of the stones and dissolves the stones. It has been used for centuries by American Indians.

There have not been enough scientific data to support or reject this herb. Safety is not known, and more research is needed to determine this herb's safety.

Juniper

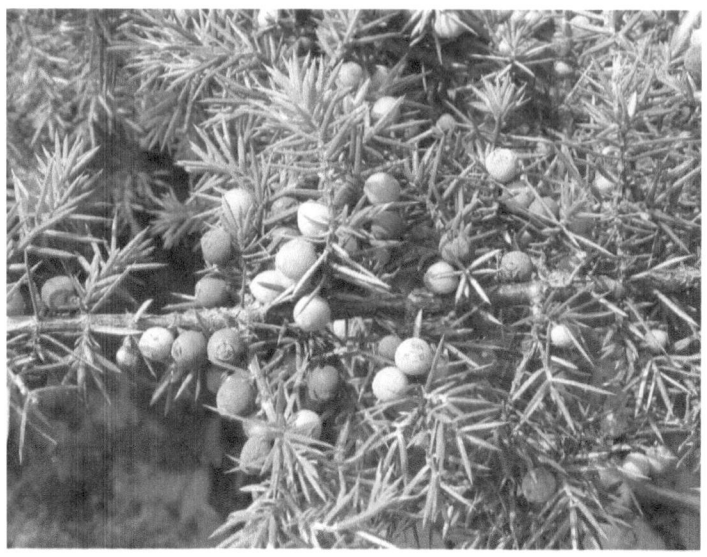

This evergreen plant is the principal flavoring for a commonly used alcoholic beverage, gin. The aromatic blue green berries have also been used in herbal medicine for centuries. It is useful for kidney stones and urinary tract infections. It can help to excrete uric acid from the body, which is important for gout management and prevention of kidney stone formation.

It is a natural diuretic. The diuretic action of the juniper is attributed to terpinene-4-ol, which increases the kidney filtration rate.

Safety of this herb is not known. More research is needed to determine safety and efficiency of this herb. High doses can cause bladder irritation.

Herbs That Improve Incontinence by Cleaning the Urinary Tract and Increasing Urination

Dandelion

The dandelion's name comes from the French *dent de lion*, or "lion's tooth" because of the toothed edges of its leaves. The entire plant is considered medicinal. Dandelion is used for kidney and bladder stones and urinary tract infections. In folk medicine, dandelion is also used as a remedy for hemorrhoids, gout, and other skin conditions. This herb has been used for many centuries. It is a natural diuretic, washing out excess water from body, soothing inflamed breast tissue.

Dandelion juice is popular for its diuretic action. It is also used for constipation and arthritis. This herb helps to eliminate uric acid from body. It can be used as a tea or tincture.

Safety is not known. More research needed to determine safety of this herb.

Parsley

Parsley originated in the Mediterranean region. The ancient Greeks held it sacred for the realms of dead. It is now growing everywhere and is a very popular garnish for cooking. This familiar garnish provides urinary system nutritional support and contains apiol. Apiol is a volatile oil that is urinary tract antiseptic. Parsley also supplies chlorophyll that helps urinary tract healthy function. It is helpful in urinary incontinence and bladder infection. Parsley contains high amounts of vitamin C.

Parsley can be consumed as tea, as dry extract, or as juice.

Safety for high doses is not known. More research is needed to establish safety and efficacy. Avoid excessive amount if you are pregnant or lactating.

Herbs That Improving Incontinence Caused by Prostate Enlargement

Pygeum

The bark of the African plum tree has been used in Africa and Madagascar traditionally for the discomfort of benign prostatic hypertrophy (BPH) and generalized urinary tract troubles and infections for centuries. The hydrocyanic acid content has a pleasant almond flavor and used for drinking and cooking.

Use

Pygeum extract is a very popular treatment for symptoms of benign prostatic hypertrophy. Botanical worldwide demand for pygeum has increased so much that it was reported that the tree was a threatened species.

How it works?

Pygeum causes a slight decrease in levels of testosterone and prolactin. It decreases in the excitability of the detrusor muscle and has antiestrogenic effects that block hyperplasia. It also increases prostatic secretions, which helps with the irritation of urethra.

Safety

Toxicity is not reported, but more research is needed for determination of safety of this herb.

Saw Palmetto

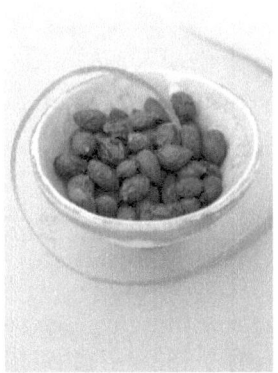

Saw palmetto, also known as *Serenoa repens* or *Sabal serrulatum*, is an herb that is taken from a partially dried ripe fruit of American dwarf palm tree, which is native in the southern coastal United States. It was widely used under the name *Serenoa* until World War II; then it was forgotten and then rediscovered in the '90s. It is most commonly used to treat problems related to benign prostatic hyperplasia.

Saw palmetto's active part is the sterols and free fatty acids found in the berry. The particular solvent used in the extraction process affects the resulting formulation of the product. It is unclear which components are the most active. This herb has anti-inflammatory activity; it also blocks conversion of testosterone to dihydrotestosterone (DHT) and may cause involution of prostate epithelial tissue.

Saw palmetto is an effective treatment for the symptoms of benign prostatic hypertrophy. It is as effective as medications and is better tolerated, less expensive.

Safety: No report of serious toxicity or adverse affects. More research is needed for long-term safety determination.

Nutritional Supplements That May Be Helpful

Bromelian (from pineapple) and trypsin may enhance the effectiveness of antibiotics in people with urinary tract infection.

D-Mannose attach to the bacteria and prevent them from attaching to the lining of urinary tract. More research and study needed for safety and efficacy of this supplement.

Vitamin C can inhibit the growth of *E. coli*. It is an antioxidant and improves healthy growth of the tissue. It also creates an unfriendly environment for bacteria in the urinary tract.

Vitamin A deficiency increases the risk of many infections. It is an important part of immune system.

Zinc plays an important role in the immune system and cell production and wound healing. It can be helpful in alleviating symptoms of enlarged prostate.

Magnesium has long year's in the history of healing. Magnesium is very important in neuromuscular contractions; it has been helpful in easing kidney stone symptoms.

Chapter Eleven

How Do I Cope with Incontinence?

Until your body responds to treatments, there are many ways to cope with incontinence. We would mention a few of these self-care ways. Be creative; you can find many effective options.

What Is a Toilet Substitute?

If you have difficulty to access the bathrooms or have frequent nighttime urgency and there is risk of fall, you may consider using toilet replacements.

You may want to use a bedside commode placed near your bed. Choose those having a grab bar that fit to your weight and height and those with a large soft surface. Disadvantages of commodes are poor support and possible instability.
You may choose to use a urinal. Urinals are more effective and easier to use in men than women.

Foley Catheter

Sometimes Foley catheter is recommended for managing urinary incontinence. Its use is usually temporary.

Foley catheter is a thin soft plastic or rubber tube that is inserted into the bladder via the urethra to drain the urine. The catheter is connected to an external bag (the external bag can be small and worn under the pants or skirts or can be large and hang from the bed). Urinary catheters are used to manage urinary incontinence and urinary retention in both men and women. There are different types of catheters, and they have different uses.

Complications

Complications of catheter use are urinary tract infections, skin irritation, urethral damage, bladder stones, and blood infection.

Catheters come in different sizes: 12 Fr, 14 Fr, 16 Fr, 30 Fr, and they are made of different materials such as Teflon, latex, and silicone. Commonly, a size 14 Fr or size 16 Fr catheter is used. It is better to use a smaller size catheter due to less injury to the urethra.

How Do I Care for My Catheter?

- Clean your urethral area (where the catheter exits the body) with soap and water.
- Clean the catheter with soap and water.
- After bowel movements, clean the perineal area to prevent spread of colonial bacteria.

How Do I Care for My Drainage Bag?

- The drainage bag should stay lower than the bladder (you do not want urine to go back into the bladder).
- Empty the drainage bag when the device is full or every 6-8 hours.
- Clean the outlet valve with soap and water if it becomes dirty.
- Wash your hands before and after handling the drainage bag.
- Clean the drainage bag periodically. You can remove the drainage bag from the catheter and place another bag during cleansing. Clean the bag with chlorine or by filling 2 parts vinegar and 3 parts water and wait for 30 minutes. Then dry the bag.

Suprapubic Catheter

A suprapubic catheter is a catheter that is placed directly into the bladder through the abdomen. The name comes from the location of the catheter that is above the pubic bones. Usually a physician places the catheter.

Complications

Urinary tract infections are more prevalent in people with urinary catheter. Make sure to inform your physician if you have any fever, chills, swelling, redness, and pain.

What is an External Catheter System?

If you are a man and confined to a wheelchair or bed and have moderate to severe incontinence, you may want to try an external catheter system also called condom catheter or penile sheaths. The advantages are less possibility of infection and less discomfort to urethra comparing to Foley catheter. The disadvantages are urinary leakage and difficulty in placing and removing it. You may need to ask a caregiver to help you.

What is an External Compression Devices (Penile Clamp)?

An external compression device or penile clamp is a device that is placed halfway down the shaft of the penis and compresses the urethra. It prevents urine leakage due to stress urinary incontinence or after prostate surgery or continuous urinary leakage. When the clamp is closed, it should stop urine flow without discomfort.

If you use a penile clamp, you should be very cautious and have good penile sensation. You should release the clamp every 2 hours to promote circulation. If you notice any color change in the penis, open the clamp immediately.

Complications

If you leave the clamp too long or if it is very tight it can cause the following:

- Circulation problems
- Skin breakdown
- Swelling
- Urethral strictures (scars inside of the urethra)

How Do I Care for My Skin?

If you experience urinary or bowel incontinence you are at great risk for skin breakdown, ulcers, and infection, especially if you are not moving and are restricted to a bed or wheelchair. If you use diaper, your skin would have continuous contact with urine and feces. Your skin becomes irritated, and skin breakdown starts. Usually the first sign is redness of the area. You should give extra care to keep skin clean and dry. Beware of skin cuts caused by tight diapers or because of tapes used. Clean the skin of the perineal area after each incontinence incidence.

You have several options for cleaning the area.

- You may want to simply clean the skin with a mild soap and water, rinse, and gently dry the area. You may apply nonalcohol moisturizing creams to keep the skin moist.
- You may use incontinence skin cleaners specifically made for the perineal area. These products clean the area without causing the skin dryness or irritation.
- You may use disposable wipes.
- You may use creams that act as skin barriers to protect skin from irritation of urine or feces.
- Be careful about yeast infection. If you suspect yeast infection (redness and rash over the skin, itchiness, and discomfort), contact your physician. You may also use antifungal creams or powders over the perineal area.

Absorbent Products

If you want to use absorbent products, choose them according to the severity of your urine leakage, your comfort, cost, ease of use, odor control, environmental effects, and your personal preferences.

You have different options.

- You may want to use perineal pads or panty liners if you have mild leakage.
- You may choose protective underwear, undergarments, or diaper-style products or adult briefs if you have for moderate to heavy leakage.

- If you are a man, you are lucky that you can use guards and drip collection pouches.
- You may use under pads for furniture and bed protection.
- Be creative. You can make extraordinary absorbent materials yourself.

Chapter Twelve

Exercises

Why Exercise the Pelvic Muscles?

Life's events can weaken pelvic muscles. Pregnancy, childbirth, and being overweight, chronic cough, smoking, and many other conditions can weaken your pelvic muscle. You can make them strong again by exercising them. Pelvic floor exercises are one of the most important and most effective ways to prevent and cure incontinence.

In our book to prevent and cure incontinence, we illustrate how to effectively and correctly do these pelvic exercises. A DVD that would show you the exercises and guide you in every step accompanies the book.

Pelvic floor muscles are like other muscles that become weak if they are untrained or are not exercised. You cannot see these muscles as you can see your deltoid and bicep muscles, so identifying them is harder and needs more time and dedication.

Once you successfully identified your pelvic muscle and started your exercises regularly, you would enjoy a strong and healthy pelvic floor. You would prevent or cure incontinence and would enjoy more satisfying sexual life for both you and your partner.

The pelvic muscles work to control the release of urine.

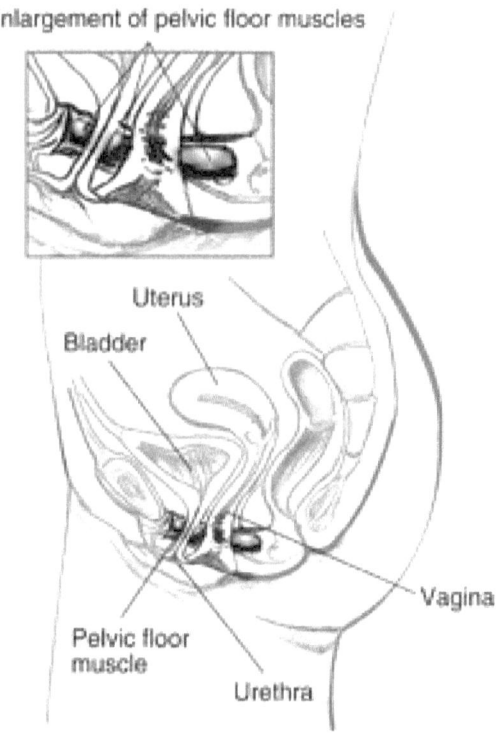

Enlargement of pelvic floor muscles

Uterus

Bladder

Vagina

Pelvic floor
muscle

Urethra

Index

www.ingramcontent.com/pod-product-compliance
Lightning Source LLC
Chambersburg PA
CBHW022129170526
45157CB00004B/1804